NATURAL THERAPY OF CYSTIC FIBROSIS

Prevention of bronchial plugging and superinfection

Constantin Panow

COPYRIGHT 2016

All rights reserved.

DISCLAIMER

The author and publisher decline responsibility about any harm or deleterious effect, which can result from wrong understanding and interpretation of following text.

This booklet is meant for information purposes alone.

Consult with your physician and dentist before applying methods described below.

CONTENT

Copyright 2016

Disclaimer

Personal history

Encouraging news

Practice

Infection

Staphylococcus aureus

Physiopathology

Nemesis

Antibiotics

History

Pasteur

Interpretation

Evolution

Factory

Less known

You would ask:

Cleaning

Other drawbacks

Resistance

Toothpaste
Science
Washing method
Negative effect
One solution
Antidry
Mouth
Sugar
Vitamin B12
Extra advice
Fruit
Ajrjian
Probiotics
Marketplace
Alcohol
Lungs
Factor Time
Website

"Nature is the best physician!"
  Hippocrates (460-370 BC)

PERSONAL HISTORY

As a medical practitioner with only one year training in lung medicine, I have been little exposed to patients with this disease.

Cases were few, but psychological imprints in my memory remain still vivid.

Lot is known about genetics of disease, fortunately autosomal recessive, but treatments remain still limited in most instances to antibiotics.

ENCOURAGING NEWS

Now a new therapy has emerged from the US, but which is still expensive, and hence limited in use.

PRACTICE

Recent evolution of medicine allows lung transplantation as last resort, but donors are exceptional and taking anti-rejection medication for the rest of one's days is not a rejoicing perspective.

What a medical doctor learns in everyday life, is how to contain disease and its complications, infectious manifestations, to a minimum.

Antibiotic therapy, physical lung treatment with the physiotherapist, and so forth, are well known topics.

This is not the aim of my short publication.

INFECTION

Recent advances in Infectious Diseases have made for us better understandable topics of physiopathology and involved pathogens.

Medical practitioners and laboratory technicians unfold little by little secrets of Nature.

STAPHYLOCOCCUS AUREUS

First, about 20 years ago appeared articles about intra-cellular survival of this bug, in sinus cavities of the head.

We understood little at that time what it meant.

Long before, we knew that this germ was responsible for skin diseases, especially acne vulgaris.

Since years appeared the term of epidermal inclusion cyst for those tortuous sebaceous glands, which is nothing else than skin caught around a hair follicle.

And you would ask why?

Because of thick secretion!

Produced by this same bacterium.

Now we know that it is one of first pathogens found in young children with complications of cystic fibrosis.

It is also prevalent in adults with this disease.

PHYSIOPATHOLOGY

Thickening of secretions for which cystic fibrosis is known allows Staphylococcus aureus an excellent medium for proliferation, with further inspissating of this provoking mucus plugging in small and medium bronchi.

NEMESIS

If this is the only problem, you would ask, why not treating every patient with this inherited disease with antibiotics as a prevention?

Well, it has been tried with negative effects for involved subjects.

You would ask why?

Because Staphylococcus aureus has a friend fighting in the camp of molds.

And mushrooms proliferate as soon you give an antibiotic.

ANTIBIOTICS

Those are produced by yeasts and similar germs to contain proliferation of bacteria.

The topic we are talking about now is called Aspergillus fumigatus, for the most prominent one, and it also stiffens bronchial secretions with production on the long run of bronchiectasis (widening of bronchial tree), with only difference that it involves bigger bronchi.

(Than the ones of cystic fibrosis).

HISTORY

To understand the meaning of nowadays prevalence of Staphylococcus aureus in so many folders of our Medicine workup, we must address previous exposure of Human Psychology to Infectious Diseases.

Optical microscopy evolved long ago and first such devices are from 17th century.

PASTEUR

Germs could be observed thus 3 centuries ago, but it is not until the end of 19th century that our great-grand parents became aware of this component of their surroundings.

INTERPRETATION

First retained and for long time imprinted meaning in our psychology is: Infectious Diseases, as it remains today!

"What is written once with ink, cannot be uprooted with an axe."

Germ=Disease!

Stressing on negative connotation!

This is the meaning which remains in general population, even nowadays!

EVOLUTION

Such a philosophy is of course without consideration for our more ancient history and the fact that all life on this Planet comes from those minute existing beings.

Well, half a century ago, a Nobel price was granted for pertaining that all life was once genetic.

But a gene is again another fairy tale like the Bible and the story of 7 days.

Now specialists consider seriously the possibility of minute germs smaller than viruses, and which have no genetic material whatsoever, but resemble proteins: the so-called prion.

FACTORY

And you would ask:

What was the result of this philosophy?

Of course, you know, the story of Alexander Fleming and how he discovered penicillin.

And since, huge Pharmaceutical Industry is trying to reinvent this success tale.

But, as you would notice remakes become less and less visited in theaters, as at the end everybody becomes bored.

Before that Mother Nature has invented germ-resistance!

LESS KNOWN

Ok. Penicillin and all other antibiotics, we all need them from time to time... A facet you would less recognize in all this fallacy soup, is the one of soaps.

Everybody washes today with soap! Or at least shampoo! Even our clothes are treated this way.

YOU WOULD ASK:

What is the result on environment? Guess twice! Our blue-green Planet is morbid. And us too!

Soaps are between the most potent antimicrobials on Earth.

CLEANING

They spare you a warm pleasant bath in the morning. No need for hot water! No vigorous rubbing necessary!

They allow for a short lukewarm showering without any exercise!

OTHER DRAWBACKS

As a result, your neighbor in the bus is still half asleep. Your underarm is stinking again in the afternoon.

And you need deodorant to keep up with your working day schedule.

RESISTANCE

Staphylococcus aureus is the only germ able to survive those potent skin solvents, which are soaps and shampoos!

TOOTHPASTE

But mouth bactericides are not an exception.

Staphylococcus aureus is not only main constituent of dental plaque, as we already know, but it could be also its first promoter.

SCIENCE

The part of proof about efficiency of cleaning oneself without soaps is simple.

Already my professor in Medical School 40 years ago showed us results of his experiments in hygiene.

He used an amazingly simple, but efficient material for this analysis.

Petry boxes, which he scraped with the hands of his staff, before washing, and after cleaning with soap or water alone.

WASHING METHOD

Soap was superior in this experiment over water alone for only 1 %.

At that time, he was mentioning this research for another purpose.

Establishment, which always has the upper hand in university, as elsewhere, imposed extremely aggressive detergent in all lavatories in University Hospital of Geneva.

NEGATIVE EFFECT

Guess the result of those products.

Small fissures and wounds on hands of all people involved in this msyophobia therapy. And as soon as the skin was no more intact, nothing could prevent growing of bacteria on it!

And on thus scraped Petry boxes!

ONE SOLUTION

And you would ask: What is the alternative?

Reinventing the old way of Native Americans, who pretended that we are part of Nature and should live our lives in harmony with it, rather than against it!

Greeks of Old and our ancestors used oil, olive oil for instance to rub one's skin.

A natural sponge or brush also possibly from non-synthetic material would do.

Essential for this type of washing is a bath, a warm bath which would dissolve the oily material.

And vigorous rubbing too! Personally, I prefer to wash with diluted Yoghurt, my nose inclusive.

If you have long and thick hair, you can replace your shampoo with vinegar, or wine.

ANTIDRY

This almond oil is sold in pharmacies in Switzerland and widely prescribed by doctors since years.

MOUTH

For this part of your body, you can produce your own toothpaste out of oil and abrasive material.

I chose sunflower oil, added one volume to one to talc, which does the job. Talc is the softest mineral, with level 1 on Mohs hardness scale, and one can scratch it with one's nail.

But there have appeared more replacements of toothpaste on Internet.

One of them is composed of ashes. (Wood-ashes)

Using an electrical toothbrush would help the extra rubbing needed.

I would advise to double cleaning time and have a regular checking with your dentist.

SUGAR

Discarding all sweets from one's regime is essential to prevent tooth holes. Consider ketogenic diet, if you like it, as this would take away further risk of caries!

Apart from that avoiding lectins and consuming gluten-free could help you tremendously.

VITAMIN B12

Adding it to this self-made toothpaste would prevent gum irritation, and to big extent plaque deposition.

As to practical advice, I add two vials (two thousand microg) to 50 g Talc (1.76 oz), mixed it with vegetal oil till consistency like toothpaste.

Tumors

Recent publications disclose association of gynecological cancer with talc use. On the opposite side, there has been no increase in lung carcinoma ratio between miners.

Since more than half a century are known cases of such neoplasia in silicosis. Reason was unclear at that time.

Now we know about co-occurrence of asbestos and silica. Such an information makes all abrasive material, and thus most toothpastes suspect.

There are reports about carcinogens in burnt food.

Hence, if you want to stay on the safe side, brush your teeth only with water. Yoghurt, vinegar, and wine would also be good.

EXTRA ADVICE

Still little used medicine in cystic fibrosis is mucous softening therapy.

Acetylcysteine is known since a long time, and recent research has shown that it is much better tolerated than previously admitted.

Dosage can thus be increased without adverse effects, but with expected benefits.

FRUIT

Secretion lighteners are common in nature, especially citrus is very well known for this effect.

Lemons are most efficient but beware not to touch your teeth with their juice, as it dissolves enamel as well.

Press a lemon in a big glass and dilute it with water, before drinking it through a straw.

Oranges, pomelos, grapefruit, mandarins, clementines have comparable properties.

Small fruit, like strawberries, raspberries and blueberries contain polyphenols, antioxidants great for your general health. There are supplements on the market containing such ingredients.

AJRJIAN

I add salt and yoghurt to lemon juice diluted in water. This beverage becomes less aggressive for your teeth.

PROBIOTICS

One professor of gastroenterology in the States admitted years ago that pills claimed to contain those are inefficient. He announced this fact despite he had been prescribing them in the past. You can try to grow yourself any of those. Besides, you do not chew them, and hence they dissolve only later in your intestine.

MARKETPLACE

Probiotics with full vitality are abundant in your grocery store!

Fermented cheese is so frequent in Western Europe.

For instance, like Gorgonzola (Italy), Camembert, the blue ones, Caprice des Dieux (France), Vacherin Mont d'Or, Saint-Etienne (Switzerland), to name a few.

Yoghurt from my home country, containing Bacillus bulgaricus is especially easy to grow.

Sauerkraut is available widely in winter. You should consume it raw, bio.

You can consider adding non-specific antimicrobials to your diet, which have no side-effects and do not lead into germ resistance in your flora. Such ones are red wine (resveratrol), garlic (allicin), curcuma (curcumin), and ginger.

Personally, I drink one glass of red wine at lunch and supper, take black garlic pills, as they are devoid of smell, curcumin with piperine tablets, to attain needed amount, and ginger with cinnamon and ground black pepper in my coffee in the morning.

Those additives are efficient against viruses, bacteria, and molds and yeast as well.

ALCOHOL

Last, but not least, these beverages, without sugar content, repopulate your mouth within minutes with beneficent germs.

Beer from so many brands, available everywhere, wine, red because of resveratrol further positive properties on one's health, strong brandy like Scotch Whisky, Rakija from the Balkan, or Cognac from France.

Vinegar also would change your buccal flora instantly. Besides, it acts also as a disinfectant.

LUNGS

As you might know from Embryology, they are an expansion of the foregut.

Of course, the digestive tract is in continuity with the trachea and further the bronchial tree.

Hence, whatever you put in your mouth produces an effect in your lungs also.

FACTOR TIME

If secretion softeners work almost immediately.

Changing one's flora on skin, sinuses, nostrils, and bronchi needs weeks and months to be realized.

Bronchi are covered by a ciliated epithelium and this kind of brush is transporting all material and covering with secretions towards trachea, and from there to esophagus or mouth.

Counter-current distribution of germs needs thus longer time.

So, be patient!
Result would not disappoint you!

WEBSITE

If you have any questions, or want to share your opinion or experience, please write in my blog:

www.thenopillshealthprospect.com

www.ingramcontent.com/pod-product-compliance
Lightning Source LLC
Chambersburg PA
CBHW071829200526
45169CB00018B/1294